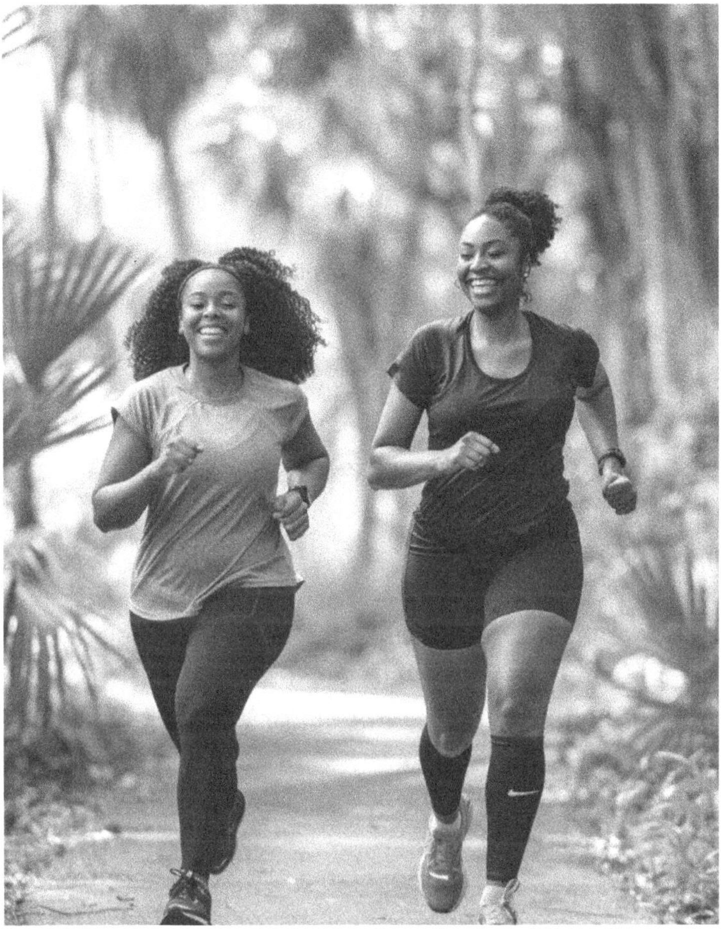

"The greatest wealth is health"

# Table of content

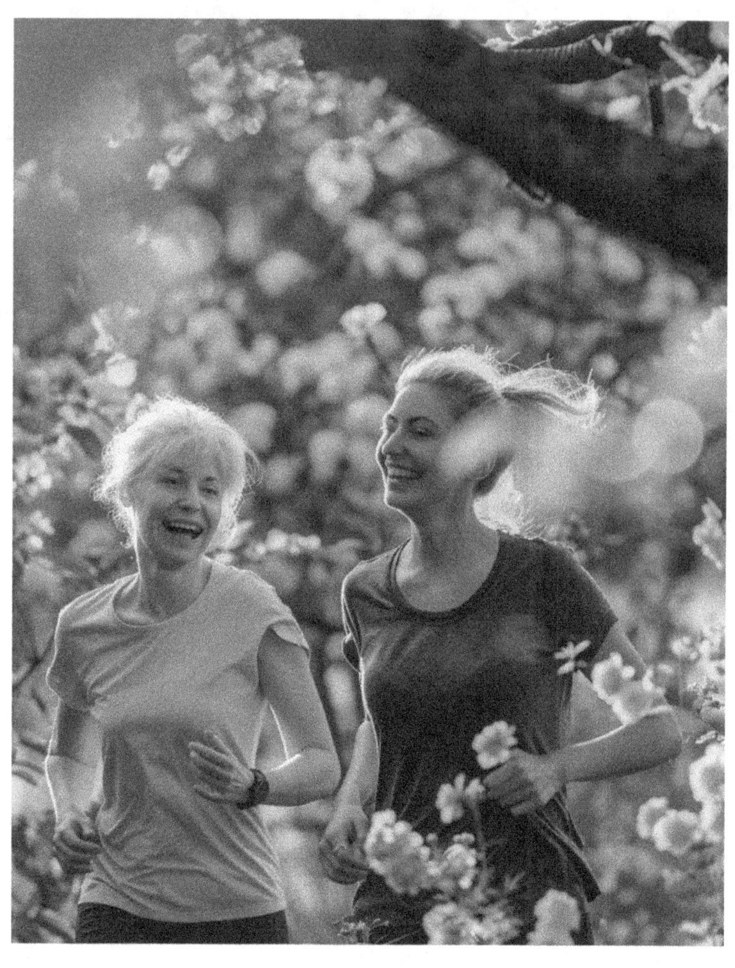

Achieving and maintaining happiness and health requires a holistic approach that addresses physical, mental, and social aspects of well-being.

# The Path to Happiness and Health: A Holistic Approach

In the modern world, the quest for happiness and health has become a central focus for many. Achieving a state of well-being involves a balanced approach that encompasses physical, mental, and social health. This article explores practical strategies to help you maintain a happy and healthy lifestyle.

**Physical Health: The Foundation of Well-being**

**1. Regular Exercise**

- **Benefits:** Improves cardiovascular health, strengthens muscles, boosts mood, and aids in weight management.
- **Recommendations:** Engage in at least 150 minutes of moderate aerobic activity or 75 minutes of vigorous activity each week, combined with muscle-strengthening exercises twice a week.
- **Tips:** Choose activities you enjoy, such as walking, cycling, swimming, or dancing, to make exercise a pleasurable part of your routine.

**2. Balanced Diet**

- **Benefits:** Provides essential nutrients, supports immune function, and maintains energy levels.

- **Recommendations:** Consume a variety of fruits, vegetables, lean proteins, whole grains, and healthy fats. Limit intake of processed foods, sugary drinks, and high-fat snacks.
- **Tips:** Plan your meals ahead of time, incorporate a rainbow of colorful fruits and vegetables, and practice mindful eating by savoring each bite.

### 3. Adequate Sleep

- **Benefits:** Enhances cognitive function, improves mood, supports physical health, and aids in weight management.
- **Recommendations:** Aim for 7-9 hours of quality sleep each night.
- **Tips:** Maintain a consistent sleep schedule, create a relaxing bedtime routine, and keep your sleep environment cool, dark, and quiet.

### Mental Health: The Key to Happiness

### 1. Stress Management

- **Benefits:** Reduces the risk of chronic diseases, improves mental clarity, and enhances emotional resilience.
- **Recommendations:** Practice mindfulness, meditation, deep breathing exercises, and yoga to manage stress.
- **Tips:** Set aside time each day for relaxation, engage in hobbies you enjoy, and avoid overcommitting to reduce stress levels.

## 2. Positive Thinking

- **Benefits:** Boosts mood, enhances problem-solving abilities, and fosters a positive outlook on life.
- **Recommendations:** Practice gratitude by acknowledging and appreciating the good things in your life. Challenge negative thoughts and replace them with positive affirmations.
- **Tips:** Keep a gratitude journal, surround yourself with positive influences, and celebrate small victories.

## 3. Social Connections

- **Benefits:** Provides emotional support, reduces feelings of loneliness, and enhances overall happiness.
- **Recommendations:** Maintain regular contact with family and friends, join social groups or clubs, and participate in community activities.
- **Tips:** Schedule regular catch-ups with loved ones, volunteer for causes you care about, and seek out new social opportunities.

## Holistic Strategies for a Happy and Healthy Life

## 1. Stay Hydrated

- **Benefits:** Supports all bodily functions, improves skin health, and aids in digestion.

- **Recommendations:** Drink at least 8 glasses of water per day, more if you are active or live in a hot climate.
- **Tips:** Carry a water bottle with you, set reminders to drink water, and consume water-rich foods like fruits and vegetables.

## 2. Limit Screen Time

- **Benefits:** Reduces eye strain, improves sleep quality, and encourages more physical activity.
- **Recommendations:** Take regular breaks from screens, especially before bedtime. Engage in offline activities like reading, exercising, or spending time outdoors.
- **Tips:** Use apps to monitor and limit screen time, designate tech-free zones in your home, and prioritize face-to-face interactions.

## 3. Practice Self-Care

- **Benefits:** Enhances self-esteem, reduces stress, and promotes relaxation.
- **Recommendations:** Make time for activities that nurture your mind, body, and soul, such as baths, reading, or nature walks.
- **Tips:** Schedule regular self-care sessions, set boundaries to protect your personal time, and explore different self-care practices to find what works best for you.

Achieving and maintaining happiness and health requires a holistic approach that addresses physical, mental, and social aspects of well-being. By incorporating regular exercise, a balanced diet, adequate sleep, stress management techniques, positive thinking, and strong social connections into your daily routine, you can create a foundation for a fulfilling and vibrant life. Remember, the journey to happiness and health is ongoing, and small, consistent efforts can lead to significant and lasting changes.

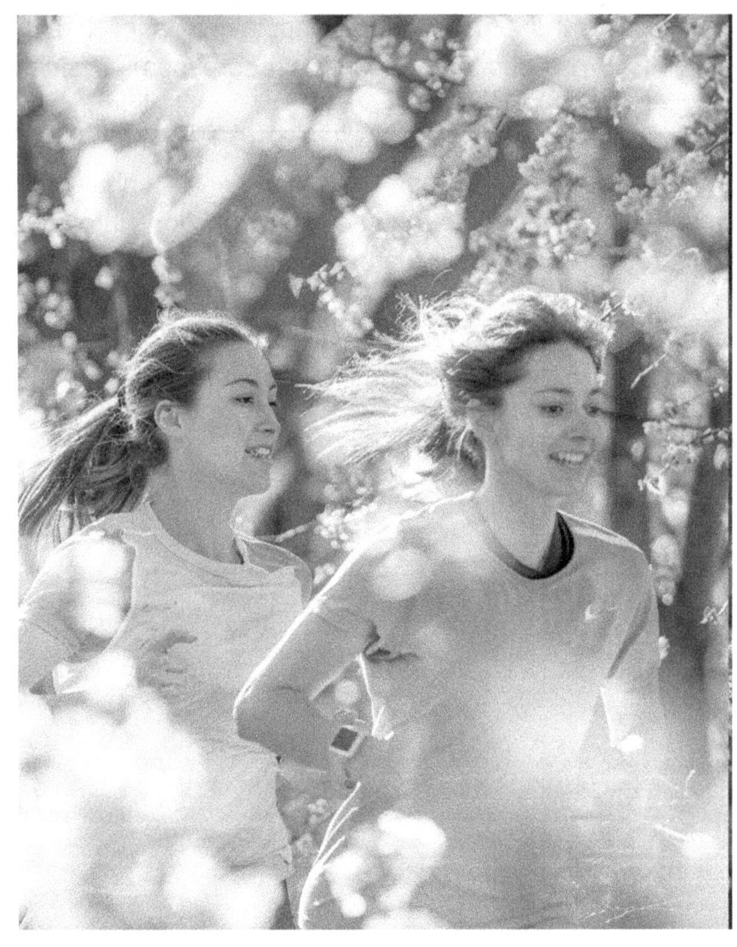

Remember, the journey to happiness and health is ongoing, and small, consistent efforts can lead to significant and lasting changes.

# The Importance of Being Healthy

In today's fast-paced world, maintaining good health has become more critical than ever. Health is not just the absence of disease but a state of complete physical, mental, and social well-being. A healthy lifestyle can lead to numerous benefits, including increased energy levels, improved mood, better sleep, and a reduced risk of chronic diseases.

**Physical Health**

Physical health is foundational to overall well-being. Regular physical activity, a balanced diet, adequate sleep, and routine medical check-ups are key components. Exercise helps maintain a healthy weight, strengthens muscles and bones, and boosts cardiovascular health. A balanced diet rich in fruits, vegetables, lean proteins, and whole grains provides essential nutrients that support body functions.

**Mental Health**

Mental health is equally important as physical health. It encompasses emotional, psychological, and social well-being. Good mental health improves productivity, enhances the ability to cope with stress, and fosters positive relationships. Practices such as mindfulness, adequate rest, and seeking support when needed are crucial for maintaining mental health.

**Social Well-being**

Social well-being refers to the ability to form satisfying interpersonal relationships and adapt to social situations. A strong social network can provide emotional support, reduce stress, and promote a sense of belonging and purpose.

## Importance of Maintaining a Healthy Weight

Maintaining a healthy weight is vital for overall health. Excess weight increases the risk of various diseases, including heart disease, diabetes, and certain cancers. Conversely, being underweight can lead to malnutrition, weakened immunity, and other health issues.

**Recommended Weight and Height Table**

To determine a healthy weight range, Body Mass Index (BMI) is commonly used. BMI is a simple calculation using a person's height and weight. The formula is:

$$BMI = \frac{Weight\ (kg)}{Height\ (m)^2}$$

Below is a table of recommended weight ranges for different heights based on BMI categories:

| Height (cm) | Underweight (BMI < 18.5) | Normal Weight (BMI 18.5-24.9) | Overweight (BMI 25-29.9) | Obesity (BMI ≥ 30) |
|---|---|---|---|---|
| 150 | < 42 kg | 42-56 kg | 57-67 kg | > 68 kg |
| 155 | < 45 kg | 45-60 kg | 61-72 kg | > 73 kg |
| 160 | < 47 kg | 47-64 kg | 65-76 kg | > 77 kg |
| 165 | < 50 kg | 50-68 kg | 69-81 kg | > 82 kg |
| 170 | < 53 kg | 53-72 kg | 73-86 kg | > 87 kg |
| 175 | < 56 kg | 56-77 kg | 78-91 kg | > 92 kg |
| 180 | < 59 kg | 59-81 kg | 82-96 kg | > 97 kg |
| 185 | < 62 kg | 62-85 kg | 86-100 kg | > 101 kg |
| 190 | < 65 kg | 65-90 kg | 91-106 kg | > 107 kg |

## Steps to Achieve and Maintain Good Health

1. **Regular Exercise**: Engage in at least 150 minutes of moderate aerobic activity or 75 minutes of vigorous activity each week, along with muscle-strengthening exercises twice a week.
2. **Healthy Eating**: Consume a balanced diet rich in fruits, vegetables, lean proteins, and whole grains. Limit the intake of processed foods, sugary drinks, and high-fat foods.

3. **Adequate Sleep**: Aim for 7-9 hours of quality sleep each night to help the body repair and rejuvenate.
4. **Stress Management**: Practice mindfulness, meditation, or yoga. Maintain a healthy work-life balance and seek support when needed.
5. **Regular Check-ups**: Schedule regular health check-ups to monitor and manage health conditions early.
6. **Hydration**: Drink plenty of water throughout the day to keep the body hydrated and functioning optimally.
7. **Avoid Harmful Habits**: Avoid smoking, excessive alcohol consumption, and drug use. These can have severe long-term effects on health.

Health is a valuable asset that requires conscious effort to maintain. By adopting a healthy lifestyle that includes balanced nutrition, regular physical activity, adequate rest, and mental wellness practices, individuals can significantly improve their quality of life. Remember, health is not a destination but a continuous journey that needs consistent attention and care.

# Recommended Healthy Foods for Weight Loss

Eating the right foods is crucial for losing weight and maintaining a healthy lifestyle. Here's a list of healthy foods that are particularly effective for weight loss:

## 1. Leafy Greens

- **Examples:** Spinach, kale, Swiss chard, collards.
- **Benefits:** Low in calories, high in fiber, vitamins, and minerals. They help increase the volume of your meals without adding calories.

## 2. Cruciferous Vegetables

- **Examples:** Broccoli, cauliflower, Brussels sprouts, cabbage.
- **Benefits:** High in fiber and protein compared to other vegetables, they help you feel full and satisfied.

## 3. Lean Proteins

- **Examples:** Chicken breast, turkey, lean beef, tofu, tempeh.
- **Benefits:** Protein increases satiety and helps preserve muscle mass during weight loss.

## 4. Fish and Seafood

- **Examples:** Salmon, trout, sardines, shrimp.
- **Benefits:** High in protein and omega-3 fatty acids, which help reduce inflammation and support metabolic health.

## 5. Whole Grains

- **Examples:** Quinoa, brown rice, oats, barley.
- **Benefits:** High in fiber and nutrients, whole grains provide sustained energy and promote a feeling of fullness.

## 6. Legumes

- **Examples:** Lentils, beans, chickpeas, peas.
- **Benefits:** High in protein and fiber, legumes are filling and help regulate blood sugar levels.

## 7. Nuts and Seeds

- **Examples:** Almonds, walnuts, chia seeds, flaxseeds.
- **Benefits:** Rich in healthy fats, protein, and fiber. They are calorie-dense but can promote satiety and support healthy metabolism when eaten in moderation.

## 8. Fruits

- **Examples:** Berries (blueberries, strawberries, raspberries), apples, oranges, grapefruit.

- **Benefits:** Low in calories and high in fiber and antioxidants, fruits satisfy sweet cravings and provide essential vitamins.

## 9. Greek Yogurt

- **Benefits:** High in protein and probiotics, which support gut health and can help you feel full longer.

## 10. Avocado

- **Benefits:** High in healthy fats, fiber, and important nutrients like potassium. Avocados can enhance satiety and reduce overall calorie intake.

## 11. Eggs

- **Benefits:** High in protein and essential nutrients. Eggs are filling and can help control appetite and calorie intake throughout the day.

## 12. Green Tea

- **Benefits:** Contains antioxidants called catechins, which may boost fat burning and metabolism.

# Sample Meal Plan for Weight Loss

**Breakfast:**

- Greek yogurt with mixed berries and a tablespoon of chia seeds.
- A slice of whole-grain toast with avocado and a boiled egg.

**Mid-Morning Snack:**

- An apple or a handful of almonds.

**Lunch:**

- Grilled chicken breast with a large mixed salad (spinach, kale, tomatoes, cucumbers) dressed with olive oil and lemon juice.
- A small serving of quinoa or brown rice.

**Afternoon Snack:**

- Carrot sticks with hummus or a small bowl of mixed berries.

**Dinner:**

- Baked salmon with steamed broccoli and roasted sweet potatoes.
- A side salad with leafy greens and a light vinaigrette.

**Evening Snack:**

- A cup of green tea and a few slices of cucumber or a small portion of Greek yogurt with a drizzle of honey.

## Tips for Success

1. **Portion Control:** Be mindful of portion sizes to avoid overeating, even with healthy foods.
2. **Hydration:** Drink plenty of water throughout the day. Sometimes thirst is mistaken for hunger.
3. **Balanced Diet:** Ensure each meal includes a mix of protein, healthy fats, and complex carbohydrates to maintain energy levels and satiety.
4. **Avoid Processed Foods:** Limit consumption of processed foods, sugary snacks, and beverages.
5. **Consistent Meals:** Try to eat meals and snacks at consistent times each day to regulate hunger and metabolism.

By incorporating these healthy foods into your diet and following balanced meal plans, you can support your weight loss goals while ensuring you get the necessary nutrients to stay healthy and energized.

# Simple and Easy Workout Plan for Weight Loss

Here's a simple and easy workout plan for weight loss, designed for a week. It includes a mix of cardio, strength training, and flexibility exercises. Always remember to warm up before starting and cool down after each workout.

## Day 1: Cardio

**Warm-up:**

- 5 minutes of brisk walking or marching in place.

**Workout:**

- 20 minutes of jogging or brisk walking.
- 10 minutes of cycling or jump rope.

**Cool-down:**

- 5 minutes of stretching (focus on legs and arms).

# Day 2: Strength Training (Upper Body)

**Warm-up:**

- 5 minutes of arm circles and light jogging.

**Workout:**

- Push-ups: 3 sets of 10-15 reps.
- Dumbbell Rows: 3 sets of 10-15 reps per arm.
- Bicep Curls: 3 sets of 10-15 reps.
- Tricep Dips: 3 sets of 10-15 reps.

**Cool-down:**

- 5 minutes of stretching (focus on arms and
  shoulders).

### Day 3: Cardio

**Warm-up:**

- 5 minutes of brisk walking or high knees.

**Workout:**

- 20 minutes of brisk walking or jogging.
- 10 minutes of jumping jacks or dancing.

**Cool-down:**

- 5 minutes of stretching (focus on legs and hips).

# Day 4: Strength Training (Lower Body)

**Warm-up:**

- 5 minutes of leg swings and light jogging.

**Workout:**

- Squats: 3 sets of 15-20 reps.
- Lunges: 3 sets of 10-15 reps per leg.
- Leg Press (if available): 3 sets of 10-15 reps.
- Calf Raises: 3 sets of 15-20 reps.

**Cool-down:**

- 5 minutes of stretching (focus on legs and glutes).

# Day 5: Cardio

**Warm-up:**

- 5 minutes of brisk walking or marching in place.

**Workout:**

- 30 minutes of any cardio activity (e.g., swimming, running, cycling).

**Cool-down:**

- 5 minutes of stretching (full body).

# Day 6: Full Body Strength Training

**Warm-up:**

- 5 minutes of dynamic stretching or light jogging.

**Workout:**

- Burpees: 3 sets of 10 reps.
- Plank: 3 sets of 30-60 seconds.
- Mountain Climbers: 3 sets of 20 reps.
- Deadlifts: 3 sets of 10-15 reps.

**Cool-down:**

- 5 minutes of stretching (focus on major muscle groups).

## Day 7: Rest or Active Recovery

### Options:

- Light yoga or stretching for 30 minutes.
- A leisurely walk for 30-60 minutes.

### General Tips:

- **Hydration:** Drink plenty of water throughout the day.
- **Nutrition:** Eat a balanced diet with plenty of fruits, vegetables, lean proteins, and whole grains.
- **Consistency:** Stick to the plan and try not to skip workouts.
- **Listen to Your Body:** If you feel pain (not to be confused with discomfort), stop and rest.

This plan is a good starting point. Adjust the intensity and duration of the exercises as needed to match your fitness level.

# Conclusion

The keys to a fulfilling life are maintaining both happiness and health. Achieving this balance involves nurturing physical health through regular exercise, a balanced diet, and adequate sleep, while also fostering mental well-being through stress management, positive thinking, and strong social connections. By embracing a holistic approach to well-being, you can create a vibrant, joyful life where health and happiness thrive together. Remember, consistent, small efforts in these areas can lead to profound, lasting changes, paving the way for a life of fulfillment and vitality.